Vegan (

**70 Of The Best Ever 1
Recipe**.......................

Samantha Michaels

Table of Contents

Cilantro Edamame Hummus
Veggie Pate
Five Pepper Hummus
Eggplant Antipasto
Magaricz
Spicy Bean Dip
Cashew Mayonnaise

Samantha Michaels

MORE 70 BEST EVER RECIPES EBOOKS REVEALED AT MY AUTHOR PAGE:-

CLICK HERE TO ACCESS THEM NOW

Publishers Notes

Disclaimer

This publication is intended to provide helpful and informative material. It is not intended to diagnose, treat, cure, or prevent any health problem or condition, nor is intended to replace the advice of a physician. No action should be taken solely on the contents of this book. Always consult your physician or qualified health-care professional on any matters regarding your health and before adopting any suggestions in this book or drawing inferences from it.

The author and publisher specifically disclaim all responsibility for any liability, loss or risk, personal or otherwise, which is incurred as a consequence, directly or indirectly, from the use or application of any contents of this book.

Any and all product names referenced within this book are the trademarks of their respective owners. None of these owners have sponsored, authorized, endorsed, or approved this book.

Always read all information provided by the manufacturers' product labels before using their products. The author and publisher are not responsible for claims made by manufacturers.

© 2013

Manufactured in the United States of America

Introduction

Eating healthy has become almost fad and due to this more and more people are turning to vegetarian meals. The problem is that many do not know the things you can eat when you skip such things as meat and dairy in your diet to ensure you are still receiving the nutrients and vitamins your body needs. With our Vegetarian lunch recipes you will easily find that you can enjoy yummy dishes without meat and even use such things as Vegan cheese or non-dairy milk to replace these items. Some of these recipes may call for a specific type of cheese; just remember that not all vegan dishes exclude dairy products. If you wish to exclude dairy products as well, you can easily find vegan replacements.

Hope you enjoy our fast and healthy Vegetarian lunch recipes.

Chapter 1 – Salads

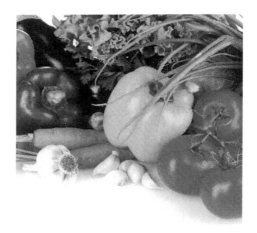

Black Bean & Veggies

Ingredients

¼ cup lime juice
¼ cup olive oil
1 tsp ground cumin
1 ½ cups cooked basmati rice
1 15oz can black beans
1 cup diced carrots
¾ cup corn kernels
¾ cup chopped tomatoes
¼ cup chopped Italian parsley
¼ cup chopped cilantro
2 tablespoons chopped red onion
Salt & pepper to taste

Preparation

In a large bowl, blend cumin, lime juice, and olive oil. Add the rest of the ingredients and stir until all are coated with the liquid mixture. Season with salt and pepper.

Samantha Michaels

Cabbage Salad

Ingredients
½ cup wine vinegar
4 tablespoon Dijon mustard
4 tablespoon sugar
½ tsp salt
12 cups shredded cabbage
10 radishes sliced
1 cup golden raisins
2 tablespoons sliced chives
Sea salt and pepper to taste

Preparation

In a bowl whisk the sugar, mustard, and vinegar. In a large bowl combine the cabbage, radishes, chives, and raisins. Once mixed pour the liquid mixture over the cabbage mixture. Toss lightly. Season with salt and pepper.

Easy Vegan Salad

Base Ingredients
Shredded cabbage
Shredded carrots
Corn
Peas
Beans
Edamame

Spices/dressing
Olive oil
Vinegar
Thyme
Oregano
Dill
Salt & pepper to taste

Add-Ins
Walnuts

Sunflower seeds
Sliced almonds
Chia seeds
Hemp seeds
Sesame seeds
Pumpkin seeds

Preparation

The best part with this recipe is that you decide what base, spices, dressing, and add ins you want to use. You create the dressing in a small bowl using the spices you desire along with either olive oil or vinegar. Once you have the dressing ready, you then get your base ready. Then add the liquid mixture and toss. Add in the other items on your add ins list and you are ready to enjoy a great salad.

Eggless Egg Salad

Ingredients

1 cup Cashew Mayonnaise (recipe on last page)
2 tablespoon chopped chives
2 tablespoon chopped parsley
3 tablespoon Dijon mustard
¼ tsp turmeric
2 pounds tofu

Preparation

In a bowl, blend all ingredients except tofu. Crumble the tofu and then gently mix. Salt and pepper to taste. Place in the refrigerator for at least 30 minutes before serving.

Lentil Orange Beet Salad

Ingredients

2 cup diced Beets
1 cup diced Orange segments
1 cup Lentils
1 head of lettuce

Preparation

Using fresh whole beets bake the night before you are going to make the salad. Wrap each beet in foil and bake for 45 minutes at 400 degrees Fahrenheit. When the beets are done, skin the beets and then dice. In a bowl, mix together the diced beets, oranges and lentils. Add the chopped lettuce and toss. Use your favorite dressing.

Mango & Grape Tomato Salad

Ingredients
2 pints of grape tomatoes
4 mangoes
½ red onion

Dressing Ingredients

1 cup mango juice
2 tablespoon lemon juice
4 tablespoons fresh mint
A tad of coriander
A tad of clove

Preparation

In a bowl, whisk together all the dressing ingredients and set aside. Cut the grape tomatoes in half, dice the mangoes, and dice the red onion. Toss these items in a bowl and then pour the dressing over the salad.

Potato Salad

Ingredients
2 ½ cup potatoes
½ cup Vegenaise
¼ cup vegan sour cream
½ clove garlic
¼ lemon squeezed
1/8 cup chopped chives
¾ tsp celery seed

Salt & pepper to taste
Paprika for garnish

Preparation

Boil the potatoes until tender, drain, and set aside to cool. In a large bowl, combine all the other ingredients while potatoes are cooling and gently mix. When the potatoes are cool, dice, and add to the mixture. Stir and sprinkle with paprika. Place in refrigerator for 2 hours before serving. Makes 4 to 8 servings.

Quinoa Sweet Potato Spinach Salad

Ingredients

2 cups Quinoa
4 cups water
4 tablespoon olive oil
2 chopped onion
4 cloves garlic (pressed)
3 cups chopped sweet potatoes
2 tsp cumin
4 handfuls of spinach leaves
4 tablespoon lemon juice
2 tablespoon tamari
2 tablespoon maple syrup
½ cup sliced almonds
Salt and pepper to taste

Preparation

In a pan, add the quinoa and water. Stir and bring to a boil, cover, and reduce heat to low. Simmer for 15 minutes. Fluff with a fork and set aside. While the quinoa is cooling, in a large skillet heat the oil on medium heat. When the oil is hot, add the garlic, onion, and sweet potatoes. Sauté until the sweet potatoes are tender. Add the cumin and cook for another two minutes and set aside. Toast the almonds over medium to low heat for about 8 to 10 minutes. In a large bowl, whisk the tamari, lemon juice, and maple syrup. Add the spinach and toss. Add the quinoa, nuts, and sweet potato mixture and combine gently. Salt and pepper to taste.

Samantha Michaels

Tabouli

Ingredients

2 bunches finely chopped parsley
1 bunch finely chopped mint leaves
1 large diced tomato
½ fined diced white onion
¼ cup cracked wheat
¼ cup lemon juice
3/8 cup olive oil

Preparation

Rinse the cracked wheat and set aside. In a bowl, add the mint, onion, parsley, and tomatoes. Add salt and pepper to taste. Combine the olive oil, lemon juice, and cracked wheat and blend well.

Tahini Kale Salad

Ingredients

2 large bunch of kale
2 15 oz can of chickpeas
2/3 cup pine nuts
1 cup sesame tahini
4 small minced cloves
3 tablespoon apple cider vinegar
2 lemons juiced
¼ cup water
Salt and pepper to taste

Preparation

Wash, trim, and dry the kale. Next, remove the stem from the kale and then chop. When finished place in large bowl. Add the chickpeas and pine nuts and mix. In another bowl add the garlic, apple cider vinegar, tahini, lemon juice, salt, and pepper and whisk. Add a little bit of water as needed until all is blended. Add the kale, beans, and pine nuts and blend well. Let stand for 15 minutes before serving.

Tuscan Bean Salad

Ingredients

2 cans Great Northern Beans (drained & rinsed)
1 cucumber cut into cubes
Red cherry tomatoes
Yellow cherry tomatoes
½ diced red onion
1 diced avocado
2 tablespoons red wine vinegar
2 tablespoons virgin olive oil
Sea salt & pepper

Preparation

Place all ingredients into a large bowl and toss gently. Add salt and pepper to taste.

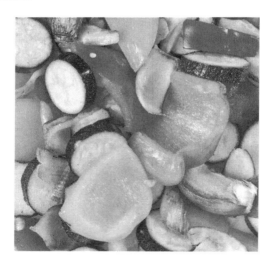

Vegetarian Greek Salad

Ingredients

2 pounds heirloom tomatoes cut into ¼ inch pieces
4 cucumbers diced
20 pitted Greek olives
8 oz cubed Greek feta
1 green pepper cut into strips

Samantha Michaels

1 red pepper cut into strips
1 yellow pepper cut into strips
1 red onion diced
6 tablespoons olive oil
½ tsp oregano
Salt & pepper to taste

Preparation

Add all ingredients into a large bowl. Toss and serve.

Chapter 2 – Soups

Potato Vegetable Soup

Ingredients

2 pounds red potatoes diced
2 onions chopped
1 10 oz package of frozen whole kernel corn
4 green peppers cut into pieces
8 minced garlic cloves
2 tsp salt
1 tsp oregano
48 oz vegetable broth
4 chopped zucchini
2/3 cup chopped cilantro

This recipe is for cooking in a crock pot. Add the potatoes, corn, onions, peppers, oregano, garlic, and salt into the crock pot. Cut all vegetables into pieces about the same size. Place all vegetables in the crock pot, cover, and cook on low heat for 7 ½ hours or 3 ½ hours on high heat. Steam the zucchini prior to putting in the crock pot and wait until the crock pot has been cooking for 15 minutes on high heat. Stir in cilantro after adding the zucchini. If you prefer to cook on the stove, cook on medium until all vegetables are tender around 1 hour. Makes 8 to 10 servings.

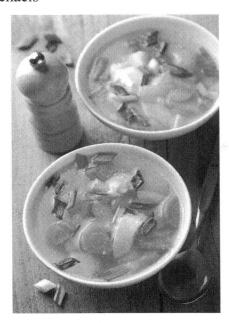

Butternut Squash Soup

Ingredients

2 butternut squash
8 cups soup stock
2 tablespoons olive oil
1 tsp cumin powder
2 tsp coriander powder
1 tsp ginger powder
½ tsp nutmeg
½ tsp cinnamon
1 tsp fennel seed powder
1 cup coconut milk
1 tsp salt
Pepper to taste

Preparation

Peel the squash and cut the ends. Remove the seeds and cut into 2 inch chunks. Add the soup stock in the crock pot with the squash. Cover and cook for 6 hours on low heat or until the squash is very tender. Take the squash out and place in a blender. Blend until smooth and set aside. Heat the olive oil in a skillet on medium low and then add the spices. Once the oil begins to bubble add the squash, coconut milk, and salt. Whisk until blended. Add the pepper to taste. Makes 12 servings.

Pinto Bean Stew

Ingredients

2 celery stalks
3 tablespoons olive oil
1 yam
½ head of cauliflower
½ tsp dried ginger
1 garlic clove
1 tsp mustard seed
½ tsp turmeric
1 tsp coriander seed
½ tsp cumin seed
½ tsp ground fennel
1 tsp paprika
2 tsp dried basil leaves
2/3 cup coconut milk
2 cans pinto beans
2 cups water
1 bay leaf
½ cinnamon stick
½ tsp salt
½ tsp pepper
¼ cup chopped parsley leaves
1 tablespoon soy sauce

Preparation

In a large pan, stir the coconut milk, water, beans, cinnamon stick, and bay leaf. Heat on low. In a skillet, heat the oil. While the oil is heating, mince the ginger and garlic, cut the yam into bite size pieces, thinly slice the celery, and cut the cauliflower into bite size pieces and set aside. Add all ingredients except cauliflower, mustard seeds, soy sauce, and bean mixture, to the oil. Sauté for

10 minutes. Add the cauliflower and cook a few more minutes. Now add the bean mixture and the mustard seed. Now, add the rest of the ingredients and cook for 20 minutes, stirring often. Makes 6 servings.

White Bean Italian Style Soup

Ingredients

2 cans Great Northern beans
4 cups peeled, cubed potatoes
2 sliced fennel bulbs
4 diced stalks celery
4 carrots, peeled and sliced
2 tablespoons olive oil
2 minced cloves garlic
2 tsp dried basil
2 tsp dried marjoram
1 tsp dried thyme
1 tsp dried ground fennel seed
1/2 tsp paprika
tad of turmeric
12 cups boiling water
2 tablespoons soy sauce pepper and salt to taste

Preparation

Heat the oil in a large pan. Prepare the vegetables. Add the garlic to the oil and sauté for a minute. Add the vegetables and sauté for 5 minutes on medium heat. Add the spices and herbs, sauté for 1 minute. Add the boiling water and cook for around 20 minutes or until vegetables are tender. Remove around 4 cups of the vegetables along with the broth, leaving the carrots. Whisk or use a mixer and blend. Pour the puree back into the soup. Drain the beans and add to soup. Cook on low for 10 minutes. Add soy sauce, salt and pepper to taste. Makes 8 servings.

Chickpea Kale Sweet Potato Stew

Ingredients

4 cups cooked chickpeas
4 cups soup stock
2 medium sweet potato chopped in bite size pieces
4 stalks celery sliced thin
8 cups chopped kale
2 tablespoon minced garlic
2 tablespoon minced ginger
2 tablespoon olive oil
2 tsp brown mustard seeds
2 tsp ground coriander seeds
1 tsp ground cumin seeds
1 tsp paprika
1 tsp ground fennel seed
1 tsp ground fenugreek seed
1 tsp turmeric
2 bay leaf
1 tsp salt or to taste
2 tsp soy sauce
Black pepper to taste
1 cup coconut milk

Preparation

In a large pot heat the beans with the bay leaf. Prepare all vegetables and spices. Heat the oil in a large skillet. Sauté the mustard seeds, ginger, and garlic for 5 minutes. Add the sweet potatoes and celery and sauté for 5 minutes. Add the spices and stir. Add the kale and stir fry until kale wilts. Add the beans, coconut milk, and liquid. Bring to a boil, cover, and cook until vegetables are tender. Add soy sauce, salt, and pepper to taste. Makes 8 servings.

Cream of Asparagus and Spinach Soup

Ingredients

2 lbs asparagus
2 lbs fresh spinach
6 cups water
2 unsalted vegan bouillon cube
2 tablespoon olive oil

4 Tablespoon flour
4 cups unsweetened soy milk.
4 Tablespoon cashew butter
½ tsp nutmeg
Pepper and salt to taste

Preparation

Prepare asparagus by cutting and discarding bottom stems and chopping into 1 inch pieces. Wash and chop the spinach removing the stems. In a large pot bring the water and bouillon cube to a boil. Reduce heat, cover, and simmer. In another large pot heat the oil on medium heat. Add the flour and stir until crumbly. Add the milk and whisk until the mixture begins to thicken. Steam the asparagus in another pan for around 5 minutes in just a small amount of water until tender. Add the spinach to the asparagus and steam until spinach wilts. Place spinach and asparagus in a blend and add 2 cups of the liquid along with the butter. Blend until smooth. Add the greens back to the soup and heat for 5 minutes on medium heat stirring constantly. Do not let the soup boil. Add the seasonings and herbs. Makes 8 servings.

Cream of Broccoli Soup

Ingredients

6 cups broccoli stalks and florets
8 cups unsalted vegetable soup stock
1 cup chopped parsley
1 tsp powdered dried rosemary
2 tsp dried powdered dried thyme
4 tablespoon olive oil
4 tablespoon chick pea flour
4 cups unsweetened rice milk
Salt & pepper to taste

Preparation

Prepare broccoli by peeling the stems and chopping into small pieces. Chop parsley and set aside. Take out 2 tablespoons to use as garnish. Place the broccoli into the soup stock in a large pan and bring to a boil. Reduce heat and simmer around 5 minutes or until broccoli is tender. Place the broccoli, parsley, liquid, rosemary, thyme, salt and pepper in a blender or use a mixer and puree until smooth, then set aside. To make the white sauce, heat the olive oil in the pan add the flour and cook for 10 minutes on low heat. Pour in the milk and whisk until mixture begins to boil and thickens around 10 minutes. Keep whisking or the sauce will become lumpy. Add the broccoli puree and heat. Do not boil. Makes 12 servings.

Cream of Cauliflower Soup

Ingredients

2 cauliflower heads
8 cups unsalted vegetable soup
1 tsp dried rosemary
2 tsp dried thyme leaf
4 tablespoons olive oil
6 tablespoons flour
1/4 tsp turmeric
1/2 tsp ground cumin
2 tsp ground coriander
1 tsp ground ginger
4 cups plain unsweetened fortified rice milk
1/2 cup minced parsley
Salt & pepper to taste

Preparation

Prepare cauliflower by removing leaves and chopping into 2 inch pieces. Place the cauliflower into the soup stock and bring to a boil. Reduce heat, cover, and simmer for 20 minutes or until cauliflower is tender. Add the soup and parsley together in a blender and puree until smooth. Set aside. To create the white sauce, heat the olive oil in the pan add the flour and cook for 10 minutes on low heat. Pour in the milk and whisk until mixture begins to boil and thickens around 10 minutes. Keep whisking or the sauce will become lumpy. Add the broccoli puree and heat. Do not boil. Makes 12 servings.

Samantha Michaels

Pumpkin Soup

Ingredients

4 tablespoons olive oil
2 tsp coriander seeds
2 tsp cumin seeds
1 tsp ground turmeric
1 tsp mustard seeds
2 onions cut chunks
4 garlic cloves
6 cups diced pumpkin
4 quartered plum tomatoes
12 cups unsalted vegetable stock
2 tablespoon lemon juice
Cilantro leaves to garnish
Pumpkin seeds to garnish
Whipped tofu to garnish (recipe below)

Preparation

Preheat oven to 400 degrees Fahrenheit. In a bowl mix the spices and oil. Once blended add the vegetables and blend. Spread on a cookie sheet and roast for 30 minutes. Place this mixture once roasted in a food processor along with half the soup stock and process until smooth. Pour into a large pan with the rest of the soup stock, put in seasoning and heat until it begins to simmer. Remove from heat and add lemon juice, stir. Serve with the whipped tofu as a garnish.

Whipped Tofu ingredients include 1 pound of silken tofu, 4 tablespoons of oil, grated zest of 2 lemons, and 1 tablespoon of non dairy milk. Puree all ingredients except in the milk in a food processor until creamy and smooth. Add the milk, stir, and chill. Let chill for 1 hour.

Makes 12 servings

Red Lentil Vegetable Soup

Ingredients

2 cups red lentils
12 cups water
2 pounds yams
2 cups sliced green beans (fresh)
4 stalks diced celery
1 diced red pepper
2 tablespoon olive
4 slices fresh ginger
1 cinnamon stick
1 bay leaf
1 tsp ground fennel
1 tsp cumin seed
2 tsp ground coriander
1 tsp turmeric
Tad of hing
Salt & pepper to taste
Garnish – 2 tablespoon parsley, cilantro, or basil.

Preparation

Prepare the lentils by cleaning, washing, rinsing, and draining. Then add the lentils to the water in a large pot and bring to a boil. Skim the foam as needed. Cover and simmer for 30 minutes. While the lentils are boiling, prepare the rest of the vegetables and set aside. Heat the oil in skillet and add hing. Add the vegetables and sauté on med/high heat for 5 minutes. Add the spices and sauté 1 minute. Remove from heat. Add the lentils and the water, ginger slices, cinnamon stick, and bay leaf. Bring to a boil, cover, and simmer 30 minutes. Add salt and pepper to taste. Makes 12 servings.

Pasta Bean Soup

Ingredients

4 cans garbanzo beans
6 cups vegetable stock
3 cups dry pasta
4 – 6 tablespoons olive oil
4 minced garlic cloves
Dash cayenne pepper
½ cup chopped parsley

2 tablespoon minced ginger
4 sliced celery stalks
4 sliced carrots
4 cup sliced green beans
1 chopped green
1 chopped red pepper
4 chopped plum tomatoes
2 tablespoons dried basil leaves
1/2 tsp dried thyme
2 tsp dried marjoram
4 tablespoon unsalted tomato paste
Salt & pepper to taste

Preparation

Put on a large pot of water for the pasta. Heat oil on medium low in a large pan. While the water and oil are getting ready, prepare your vegetables. To the oil, add the ginger and garlic, stir. Add the green beans, peppers, carrots, and celery. Sauté for 5 minutes on med/high heat. Add the herbs and tomatoes and sauté for 2 minutes. Add the spices and dried herbs and sauté for 1 minute. Drain the beans and add to the vegetables. Add the tomato paste and 1 cup of the liquid, cover, simmer until vegetables are tender. Cook the pasta in the boiling water for 5 minutes. When the pasta is done and the vegetables are tender add the pasta to the vegetable and bean pot. If needed add more liquid. Cook for 5 minutes. Salt and pepper to taste.

Makes 16 servings.

Beet Soup

Ingredients

4 cups grated beets
4 cups shredded red cabbage
4 diced potatoes
4 tablespoon red wine vinegar
6 diced tomatoes
½ cup vegan butter
8 cups soup stock

2 grated onions
2 grated carrots
1 tablespoon sugar
Salt and pepper to taste

Preparation

Place the beets, potato, and cabbage in a large pot with the vinegar and tomato along with half the butter and all the soup stock. Simmer for 1 hour. In another pan, melt the butter and add the onion and carrot, sauté until golden. Add this mixture to the large pot with the beets. Cover and simmer for 15 minutes. Salt and pepper to taste. Add the sugar. Makes 12 servings.

Chapter 3 – Sandwiches & Burritos

Falafel Sandwiches

Ingredients

Sauce:

1 cup Greek yogurt
1 tablespoon tahini
1 tablespoon lemon juice

Falafel:

¾ cup water
1/4 cup uncooked bulgur
3 cups cooked chickpeas
1/2 cup chopped cilantro
1/2 cup chopped green onions
1/2 cup water
2 tablespoons all-purpose flour
1 tablespoon ground cumin
1 teaspoon baking powder
3/4 teaspoon salt
1/2 teaspoon ground red pepper
3 garlic cloves
6 (2.8-ounce) Mediterranean Style white flatbreads
12 (1/4-inch-thick) slices tomato

Preparation

Prepare the sauce by combining all the ingredients and whisking until blended. Cover and chill. Prepare the falafel by bring the water to a boil and adding the bulgur. Remove from heat, cover, and let stand for 30 minutes or until bulgur is tender. Drain and set aside. Preheat oven to 425°. In a food processor add the chickpeas and the other ingredients through garlic on the list. Blend until smooth. Place this mixture in a large bowl and add the bulgur. Divide into 12 equal portions around ¼ cup each. Shape into ¼ inch patty. Place the patties on a cookie sheet and bake for 10 minutes or until brown. Spread the sauce on the flatbread; add 2 patties and 2 tomato slices. Makes 6 servings.

Asparagus Sandwich

Ingredients

2 bunch trimmed asparagus
2 quartered red bell pepper
2 tablespoon olive oil
6 hoagie rolls
12 ounces shredded Vegan cheese
2 sliced tomatoes
6 tablespoons vegan mayonnaise
6 tablespoons lemon juice
2 tsp minced garlic

Preparation

Preheat oven to 350 degrees Fahrenheit. Toss the red pepper and asparagus with the olive oil. Place on a cookie sheet and bake until tender around 10 minutes. Cool and remove the skin form the pepper and slice. Cut the hoagie rolls in half and place on a cookie sheet. Toast lightly. On one side of the hoagie put 4 to 5 asparagus spears with a few strips of pepper. Place the tomato on the other side. Sprinkle with the cheese and place in the oven for 5 minutes or until cheese is melted. In a bowl, mix the vegan mayonnaise, garlic, and lemon juice. Spread the mixture on one side of the roll, close, and enjoy. Makes 6 servings.

California Grilled Veggie Sandwich

Ingredients
½ cup vegan mayonnaise
6 minced cloves garlic
2 tablespoon lemon juice
¼ cup olive oil
2 cups sliced red peppers
2 sliced small zucchini
2 sliced red onions
2 sliced small yellow squash
2 focaccia bread sliced horizontally
1 cup feta cheese

Preparation

In a small bowl, blend the vegan mayonnaise, lemon juice, and garlic and place in the refrigerator. Prepare your grill for high heat. Spread olive oil on the vegetables and brush the grate with oil. Place the onion and squash around the them. Cook for 3 minutes, turn, and cook for 3 minutes more. Remove and set aside. Spread the vegan mayonnaise mixture on the sides of the bread and sprinkle with feta cheese. Place on the grill with the cheese up. Cover and cook for 2 minutes. Remove and layer with vegetables. Makes 8 servings.

Sweet Potato Burritos

Ingredients

1/2 tablespoon vegetable oil
½ chopped onion
2 minced cloves garlic
3 cups drained canned kidney beans
1 cup water
1 1/2 tablespoons chili powder
1 tsp ground cumin
2 tsp prepared mustard
1 1/2 tablespoons soy sauce
2 cups cooked and mashed sweet potatoes
6 warmed flour tortillas
4 ounces shredded Cheddar cheese or vegan cheese
Cayenne pepper to taste

Preparation

Preheat oven to 350 degrees Fahrenheit. Sauté garlic and onion in oil over medium heat until soft. Stir in the beans, mash, and gradually add the water. Heat until warm. Remove from heat and add the mustard, soy sauce, chili powder, cumin, and cayenne pepper. Stir until well blended. Divide the bean mixture and the sweet potatoes even between the tortillas. Sprinkle with cheese and place on cookie sheet. Bake for 12 minutes. Makes 6 servings.

Black Bean Burgers

Ingredients

2 drained cans black beans
2/3 cup chopped onion
2 tablespoon minced garlic
2 tablespoon cornstarch
2 tablespoon warm water
6 tablespoons chile-garlic sauce
2 tsp chili powder
2 tsp ground cumin
2 tsp seafood seasoning
1/2 tsp salt
1/2 tsp black pepper
4 slices whole-wheat bread in small crumbs
1 1/2 cups unbleached flour
8 hamburger buns

Preparations

Preheat oven to 350 degrees Fahrenheit. Grease a baking sheet. Mash the beans in a bowl. Add the onion and garlic. Mix well. In another bowl, whisk the chile garlic sauce, water, cornstarch, cumin, chili powder, salt, pepper, and seafood seasoning. Add this mixture to the beans and stir. Add the bread crumbs and stir. Add the flour but only 1/3 cup at a time until the mixture is a sticky batter form. Create mounds of around ¾ inch thickness and spoon into the baking pan and shape into burger. Bake for around 10 minutes until the outside is crisp. Makes 8 servings.

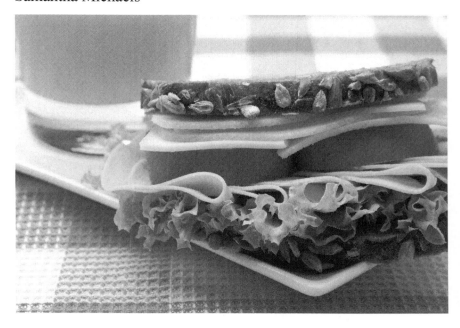

Chickpea Sandwich

Ingredients

28 oz drained garbanzo beans
2 chopped celery stalks
1 chopped onion
2 tablespoon vegan mayonnaise
2 tablespoon lemon juice
2 tsp dried dill weed
Salt and pepper to taste

Preparation

Drain and rinse the garbanzo beans. Place the beans in a bowl and mash. Add the celery, onion, dill, lemon juice, vegan mayonnaise, salt and pepper. Makes 6 servings.

Vegan Tuna Salad

Ingredients

28 oz chickpeas
4 tablespoons vegan mayonnaise

4 tablespoons spicy brown mustard
2 tablespoon sweet relish
4 chopped green onions
Salt & pepper to taste

Preparation

Combine all ingredients in a large bowl. Mix well and serve. Makes 8 servings.

Black Bean Burritos

Ingredients

4 flour tortillas
4 tablespoons vegetable oil
2 chopped onions, chopped
1 chopped red bell pepper
2 tsp minced garlic
2 15 oz can black beans
2 tsp minced jalapeno peppers
6 ounces vegan cream cheese
1 tsp salt
4 tablespoons chopped cilantro

Preparation

Preheat oven to 350 degrees Fahrenheit. Wrap the tortillas in aluminum foil and bake for 15 minutes. In a skillet heat the oil and add the jalapenos, onion, garlic, and bell pepper. Sauté for 2 minutes. Add the beans to the skillet and cook for another 3 minutes. Cut the cream cheese into pieces and add to the skillet. Stir in the salt and cook another 2 minutes. Add the cilantro and stir. Spoon mixture evenly down the center of the warm tortilla and roll. Makes 4 servings.

Zucchini Grinders

Ingredients

2 tablespoon vegan butter
4 cubed zucchini

¼ tsp red pepper flakes
Salt and pepper to taste
2 cups marinara sauce
3 cups shredded mozzarella cheese
8 split French sandwich rolls

Preparation

Preheat oven to 350 degrees Fahrenheit. In a skillet melt the butter and then fry the zucchini until a tad tender and browned. Add the salt, pepper, red pepper flakes, and marinara sauce. Stir and cook until sauce it warm. Add a spoonful of the zucchini mixture to each roll. Top with the cheese. Close the roll and wrap in foil. Bake for 15 minutes until cheese melts. Makes 8 servings.

Broiled Tomato Sandwich

Ingredients

4 tablespoons olive oil
4 tablespoons balsamic vinegar
8 sliced tomatoes, sliced
6 tablespoons vegan mayonnaise
1 tsp dried parsley
1/2 tsp dried oregano
1/2 tsp black pepper
6 tablespoons grated Parmesan cheese
8 slices toasted bread

Preparation

Preheat the oven to broil. In a bowl, whisk the vinegar and olive oil. Add the tomatoes and allow to marinate, stirring once a while. In another bowl, combine the oregano, parsley, vegan mayonnaise, 4 tsp Parmesan cheese, and pepper. Spread this mixture on the toasted bread. Add the marinated tomatoes on 4 slices of the bread and sprinkle with parmesan cheese. Place the bread on a baking sheet and broil for 5 minutes or until cheese is melted and slightly brown. Makes 4 servings.

Cucumber Sandwich

Ingredients

2 slices whole wheat bread
4 tablespoons softened cream cheese
12 slices cucumber
4 tablespoons alfalfa sprouts
2 tsp olive oil
2 teaspoon red wine vinegar
2 sliced tomato
2 leaves of lettuce
2 oz sliced pepperoncini
1 mashed avocado

Preparation

Spread each slice of bread with 1 tablespoon of cream cheese. On 2 slices of bread arrange the cucumber slices in one layer. Cover with the sprouts and sprinkle with vinegar and oil. Layer the lettuce, tomato slices, and pepperoncini. Spread the other 2 slices of bread with the mashed avocado. Close the sandwiches and serve. Makes 2 servings.

Portobello Sandwiches

Ingredients

1 clove minced garlic
3 tablespoons olive oil
1/4 tsp dried thyme
1 tablespoons balsamic vinegar
Salt and pepper to taste
2 large Portobello mushroom caps
2 hamburger buns
1/2 tablespoon capers
1/8 cup vegan mayonnaise
1/2 tablespoon drained capers
½ sliced tomato
2 leaves lettuce

Preparation

Preheat oven on broil. Adjust the rack to ensure it is close to the heat source. In a bowl, blend the thyme, olive oil, garlic, vinegar, salt, and pepper. Place the mushroom caps with the bottom side up in a shallow baking pan. Brush the caps with ½ of the dressing. Place under the broiler and cook for 5 minutes. Turn the caps and brush with the rest of the dressing. Broil 4 minutes. Toast the buns. In a bowl, mix the vegan mayonnaise and capers. Spread the mayonnaise on the buns and add the mushroom caps, lettuce, and tomato. 2 servings.

Chapter 4 – Veggie & Pasta Dishes

Pasta Primavera Recipe

Ingredients

1/4 pound angel hair pasta
1 cup broccoli florets
1/2 diced zucchini, diced
2 asparagus spears
1/4 cup peas
1/4 cup snow peas
1 1/2 minced garlic cloves
2 diced tomatoes
6 chopped basil leaves
2 tablespoon vegan butter
1/8 cup vegetable broth
¼ cup heavy cream
¼ cup grate parmesan cheese
Salt to taste

Preparation

Boil a large pot of very salted water. Boil the broccoli for 1 minute. Next and the asparagus and boil for one minute. Add the snow peas and boil for ½ a minute. Remove all the vegetables and plunge into the ice water. Once the vegetables are cool, drain. In a sauté pan, heat the butter and add zucchini and garlic. Sauté 1 minute. Add the tomatoes and sauté 2 minutes. Pour in the vegetable broth and bring to a boil on high heat. Add the cream and the vegetables. Stir. Turn the heat down and simmer. Add the cheese and stir. Cook the pasta as directed on the package. Add the pasta to the sauce. Add basil, salt, and pepper. Makes 2 servings.

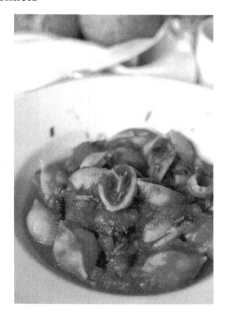

Fettuccine with Pesto Sauce

Ingredients

2 can cannelloni
2 cups basil leaves
2 tablespoons olive oil
2 tablespoons lemon juice
2 garlic cloves
6 tablespoons water
½ cup chopped walnuts
8 oz pasta
Salt & pepper to taste

Preparation

Place the garlic in a food processor and pulse until well chopped. Add the rest of the ingredients and blend until creamy usually around 2 ½ minutes. Add water when needed. Boil the pasta and pat dry. In a pan, mix ¼ cup of the sauce with the pasta. Warm and serve. Makes 4 servings.

Vegetable Orzo

Ingredients

12 oz of orzo pasta
2 diced onions
3 tablespoons olive oil
1 diced greed pepper
1 diced red pepper
1 diced squash
8 oz mushrooms
¼ cup vegan butter
1 tablespoon onion soup mix

Preparation

Cook and drain the orzo pasta. Sauté the onions in warmed oil ten minutes. Add the squash and peppers, sauté until the peppers are tender. Add the mushroom and cook until tender. Add the butter, orzo, and soup mix. Blend well. Cook for 15 minutes. Makes 8 to 10 servings.

Spicy Potato Curry

Ingredients

8 cubed potatoes
4 tablespoons vegetable oil
2 diced onions
6 minced garlic cloves
4 tsp ground cumin
3 tsp cayenne pepper
8 tsp curry powder
8 tsp garam masala
2 pieces of minced ginger root
4 tsp salt
30 oz diced tomatoes
30 oz chickpeas
30 oz peas
28 oz coconut milk

Preparation

Place the cubed potatoes in a large pot and cover with salted water bring to a oil over high heat. Reduce the heat to medium low, cover and simmer for 15 minutes. Drain and allow to seam dry for a couple of minutes. In a large skillet, heat the oil over medium heat. Add the onion and garlic. Cook and stir until the onions are soft around 5 minutes. Add the salt, ginger, curry powder, garam masala, cayenne pepper, and cumin, cook for 2 minutes. Add the potatoes, chickpeas, peas, and tomatoes. Stir and then add the coconut milk. Bring to a simmer. Simmer for 10 minutes. Makes 12 servings.

Vegan Mac & Cheese

Ingredients

I pound macaroni
2 tablespoon vegetable oil
2 chopped onions
2 cup cashews
2/3 cup lemon juice
2 2/3 cups water
salt to taste
2/3 cup canola oil
8 oz roasted red pepper
6 tablespoon nutritional yeast
2 tsp garlic powder
2 tsp onion powder

Preparation

Preheat oven to 350 degrees Fahrenheit. Bring a large pot of salted water to a boil. Pour in the macaroni and cook for around 10 minutes. Drain and place in a baking dish. In a skillet heat the oil and sauté the onion until tender and brown. Stir the macaroni into the skillet gently. In a blender add the lemon juice, salt, water, and cashews. Blend in the roasted red peppers, canola oil, garlic powder, yeast, and onion powder. Blend until mixture is smooth. Stir this mixture with the macaroni. Bake for 45 minutes or until browned on top. Makes 8 servings.

Tomato Pesto

Ingredients

4 cups basil leaves
10 sun dried tomatoes
6 crushed garlic cloves
½ tsp salt
6 tablespoons toasted pine nuts
½ cup olive oil

Preparation

In a blender, add the tomatoes, garlic, basil, salt, and nuts. Puree and then slowly add the olive oil and blend until the texture you desire. Pour over your favorite cooked pasta. Makes 6 servings.

Baked Mac & Cheese

Ingredients

6 tablespoons breadcrumbs
2 tsp virgin olive oil
1/2 tsp paprika
2 10-ounce package frozen spinach (thawed)
3 ½ cups vegan milk
6 tablespoons all-purpose flour
4 cups shredded extra-sharp Cheddar cheese
2 cups vegan cottage cheese
1/4 tsp ground nutmeg
1/2 tsp salt
Salt & pepper to taste
16 ounces whole-wheat macaroni

Preparation

Preheat oven to 450 degrees Fahrenheit. Grease a 2 quart baking dish. In a bowl, mix the breadcrumbs, paprika, and oil. In a saucepan heat 3 cups of the milk until steaming. Whisk the rest of the milk with the flour until smooth. Add this mixture to the hot milk and stir constantly until it thickens usually around 3 minutes.

Remove from heat. Add the cheese until it melts. Stir in the cottage cheese, salt, pepper, and nutmeg. Cook the pasta until dente. Drain and add to the cheese sauce until well mixed. Place half of the pasta mixture in the baking dish. Place the spinach on top of the pasta. Add the remainder of the pasta. Sprinkle with the breadcrumb mixture. Bake for 30 minutes. Makes 8 servings.

Sesame Noodles

Ingredients

1/2 pound whole-wheat spaghetti
1/4 cup soy sauce
1 tablespoon sesame oil
1 tablespoon canola oil
1 tablespoon lime juice
3/4 tsp crushed red pepper
½ sliced scallions
2 cups snow peas
1 small sliced red bell pepper
1/4 cup toasted sesame seeds

Preparation

Cook spaghetti as directed on package. Drain and rinse under cold water. Whisk the canola oil, line juice, sesame oil, soy sauce, scallions, and red pepper. Add the bell pepper, snow peas, and noodles. Toss and garnish with sesame seeds. Makes 4 servings.

Fettuccine Alfredo

Ingredients

1 ½ cups vegetable broth
8 garlic cloves
8 oz whole wheat fettuccine
2 zucchini cut into tiny slices
4 tablespoons vegan sour cream
¼ tsp pepper
1 ½ cups grated Parmesan cheese
2 tablespoon chopped parsley

4 tsp cornstarch blended with 2 tablespoons of water

Preparation

Place the garlic and broth in a sauce pan and bring to a boil over high heat. Cover, reduce heat, and allow to simmer until garlic is soft. Cook the fettuccine as directed on the package. Once the fettuccine has boiled for 8 minutes add the zucchini and cook until fettuccine is tender. Place the garlic mixture in a blender and process for 1 minute. Add the mixture back to the same pan and bring to a boil. Add the blended cornstarch and whisk until thickened around 15 minutes. Remove from heat and whisk in the pepper, nutmeg, and sour cream. Return to the pot and keep on low heat. Drain the pasta. Add the sauce and half of the parmesan cheese. Toss. Sprinkle with the remainder of the parmesan cheese and parsley. Makes 4 servings.

Orecchiette

Ingredients

3 cups of chiocciole
1 bunch chopped broccoli rabe
1 ½ vegetarian broth
4 tsp all purpose flour
2 tablespoon extra virgin olive oil
8 minced garlic cloves
¼ dried rosemary
16 oz can chickpeas (drained)
4 tsp red wine vinegar
¼ tsp salt
½ tsp ground pepper

Preparation

Cook pasta for 6 minutes in a large pot of boiling water. Add the broccoli rabe and cook until the broccoli is just getting tender which is around 3 minutes. Drain. Rinse the pot and dry. Whisk the flour and broth in a bowl. Heat the oil in skillet. Add the rosemary and garlic, cook for 1 minute. Whisk in the broth mixture. Bring to a simmer while constantly whisking. Cook until mixture thickens. Add the chickpeas, pasta, vinegar, salt, and pepper. Cook while stirring until completely heated around 2 minutes. Makes 4 servings.

Bean Bolognese

Ingredients

14 oz can of beans
2 tablespoons virgin olive oil
1 chopped onion
½ cup chopped carrots
¼ cup chopped celery
½ tsp salt
4 chopped garlic cloves
1 bay leaf
14 can diced tomatoes
¼ chopped parsley
8 ounces whole wheat fettuccine
½ cup grated parmesan cheese

Preparation

Mash ½ cup of the beans in a bowl. Heat oil in a large skillet and add onion, celery, carrot, and salt. Cover and cook until soft around 10 minutes. Add bay leaf and garlic. Cook around 15 seconds. Add wine, turn heat to high and boil until the majority of the liquid has evaporated around 3 to 4 minutes. Add tomatoes along with the juice, mashed beans, and 2 tablespoons parsley. Bring to simmering and cook while stirring until thickened around 5 minutes. Add the rest of the beans and cook another 2 minutes. While cooking this, cook the pasta as directed on package until almost tender about 8 minutes. Drain. Divide the pasta into 4 servings. Remove the bay leaf and add to the pasta. Sprinkle with Parmesan cheese and parsley. Makes 4 servings.

Asparagus Pasta

Ingredients

4 oz whole wheat penne
1 bunch asparagus cut into bite size pieces

¾ cup non dairy milk
2 tsp mustard
2 tsp flour
¼ tsp salt
¼ tsp pepper
1 tsp extra virgin olive oil
1 ½ tablespoons minced garlic
¼ tsp dried tarragon
¼ tsp grated lemon zest
1 tsp lemon juice
¼ cup parmesan cheese

Preparation

Cook pasta as directed on package for 3 minutes less than the directions on the package. Add the asparagus and cook until the asparagus is tender. Drain and return to the pot but not on the heat. Whisk the flour, mustard, milk, salt and pepper in a bowl. Heat oil in a pan over medium high heat add garlic and cook until browned around 1 minute. Whisk in the milk mixture and bring to a simmer constantly stirring. Cook until thickened around 2 minutes. Stir in lemon juice, lemon zest, and tarragon. Add the sauce to the pasta mixture. Cook, stirring constantly until sauce thickens and completely coats the pasta around 2 minutes. Stir in ¼ cup Parmesan cheese. Divide the pasta into 2 bowls and add divide the remainder of the Parmesan cheese to the 2 bowls. Makes 2 servings.

Chapter 5 - Tempeh Dishes

BBQ Tempeh

Ingredients

16 oz tempeh

2 small onions

2 cup BBQ sauce

Preparation

Cut the tempeh into 6 strips. Dice the onion. Place onion and tempeh in a shallow baking dish. Top with BBQ and marinate in the refrigerator overnight or at least 6 hours. Preheat oven to 350 degrees Fahrenheit. Cover with baking dish with foil and bake in oven for 30 minutes. Makes 6 servings.

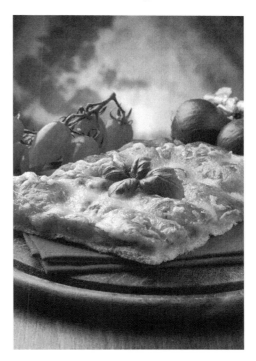

Tempeh Mexican Pizza

Ingredients

16 small corn tortillas
3 tablespoon olive oil
16 oz tempeh
2 tablespoon taco seasoning
1 tablespoon cumin
1 tablespoon garlic powder
1 cup refried beans
8 tablespoons salsa
2 cups shredded vegan cheese
2 diced tomatoes
4 sliced green onions

Preparation

Preheat oven to 400 degrees Fahrenheit. Rub a small amount of olive oil on both sides of the tortilla shells and place on baking sheet. Bake for 8 minutes, turning every 2 minutes. Now, cool oven to 350 degrees Fahrenheit. Chop the tempeh until it is the consistency of ground meat. Add a drop of water to a large skillet. Add the tempeh, garlic powder, cumin, and taco seasoning. Stir and cook until hot and all water is soaked up, stirring every once in awhile. If it begins to dry out before becoming hot add another drop of water. Place the tempeh on 8 of the tortilla shells. Spread the beans of the rest. Place them together like a sandwich. On top of each one spread 1 tablespoon of salsa. Sprinkle the cheese on top and add the tomatoes and green onions. Place on the baking sheet and bake for 3 minutes. Makes 8 servings.

Tempeh, Lettuce, and Tomato Sandwiches

Ingredients

1/2 package tempeh
1/2 cup warm vegetable broth
1 1/4 tablespoons soy sauce
1/2 tsp Liquid Smoke
1/4 tsp onion powder
1/4 tsp garlic powder

1/8 teaspoon chipotle chili powder

Preparation

Slice the tempeh around ¼ inch thick. Place the tempeh in a large skillet in a single layer. In a bowl, mix all the ingredients and pour over the tempeh. Bring to a boil, reduce heat, and simmer. Simmer for 10 minutes, turning the tempeh after 5 minutes. Remove and let sit in the broth. Get another large skillet ready by spraying with cooking spray. Heat until the skillet is hot, place the tempeh slices into the pan. Cook until brown, turn, and brown that side. Just before the bottom is brown add a couple of tablespoons of broth to the pan and allow to evaporate. Remove from pan. Place on bread with lettuce and tomato for your sandwiches. Makes 2 servings.

Roasted Corn and Tempeh Salad

Ingredients
3 cups Romaine lettuce
1 yellow tomato
1 cucumber
4 mushrooms
2 tablespoons cilantro
2 ounces of tempeh
3 tablespoons salsa
1 cup roasted corn
1 tablespoon goddess dressing

Preparation

Toss the cilantro, mushrooms, cucumber, tomato, and lettuce in a large bowl. Put in the refrigerator to chill. In a pan, sauté the roasted corn, tempeh, and salsa until thoroughly heated. Place the lettuce mixture in 2 bowls, divide the tempeh mixture and place on top of the lettuce. Top with the dressing. Makes 2 servings.

Almond Crusted Tempeh Cutlets

Ingredients

1 pound tempeh cut into slices
¼ cup almond butter
1 tsp soy sauce
¼ cup water
1 cup ground almonds
2 tablespoons peanut oil
For salsa
1 pint strawberries
1 chopped mango
1 minced jalapeno
¼ cup minced red onion
¼ cup minced red bell pepper
juice from 1 lime
¼ cup minced mint leaves

Preparation

In a medium saucepan, place the tempeh and cover with water. Bring to a simmer and allow to simmer for 10 minutes. Drain the tempeh, dry, and set aside to cool. In a bowl, add the butter and water to make a smooth batter. Put the ground almond on a flat plate. Dip the tempeh slices in the almond butter and coat with the almonds and set on another plate. Heat the oil in a large skillet. Add the tempeh and cook until lightly brown on both sides around 5 minutes per side.

For the Salsa

Chop the strawberries and place in a bowl, add the rest of the ingredients and mix well. Can be served warm or chilled. Add the mint as the last ingredient and stir gently. Makes 4 servings.

Tempeh Chicken Salad

Ingredients
½ package tempeh cubed
Small amount of water to boil tempeh
1 tablespoon olive oil
1 ½ tablespoon vegan mayonnaise
1 tsp lemon juice

Samantha Michaels

1 tablespoon minced onion
2 stalks minced celery
½ tablespoon dried parsley
1/8 tsp curry powder
Salt and pepper to taste

Preparation

Place the tempeh in a pan of boiling water, lower heat, and simmer for 15 minutes. Drain. Fry the tempeh in the oil for 5 minutes stirring often. Set aside to cool. In a large bowl, combine the tempeh with all the other ingredients. Makes 2 servings.

Tempeh Cashew Noodles

Ingredients

½ cup cashews
4 oz tempeh cubed
¼ chopped onion
1 tablespoon olive oil
1 garlic clove
2 tablespoons soy sauce
1 ½ tablespoons wine vinegar
½ tsp sugar
½ tablespoon toasted sesame oil
½ tablespoon chili paste
½ sliced zucchini
½ package of udon noodles
½ cup frozen peas

Preparation

Fry the tempeh, onion, and zucchini in olive oil until the onion is brown and soft. Boil the water for the noodles and cook according to the package. When the noodles are done, add peas. Rinse when the peas are done. In a blender, combine garlic, soy sauce, vinegar, sugar, sesame oil, chili, and the cashews. Blend until smooth and then add to the tempeh mixture. Pour this mixture over the noodles and stir. Makes 2 servings.

Italian Tempeh Nuggets

Ingredients

1 pound tempeh
Marinade:
2 tablespoons olive oil
3 tablespoons balsamic vinegar
3 tablespoons soy sauce
4 minced garlic cloves
1 tsp red pepper flakes
2 tsp dried thyme
2 tsp dried basil
2 tsp dried rosemary

Preparation

Cut the tempeh into ½ inch cubes. Combine the ingredients for the marinate in a bowl with a lid and stir. Add tempeh, put on the lid, and shake well. Chill in the refrigerator for at least one hour. Shake the container every once in awhile. Heat a skillet over medium low heat. Add the tempeh with any liquid you desire and cook for 10 minutes. Turn as cooking. Makes 2 servings.

Tempeh Salad

Ingredients

8 oz soy tempeh
1/8 cup sweet relish
1/8 cup chopped celery
1/8 cup chopped red onion
1/8 cup diced red bell pepper
1/8 cup raw sunflower seed
1/8 cup diced green pepper
1/8 cup sliced scallion
1 tablespoon tamari
1 tablespoon chopped parsley
1 tablespoon lemon juice
¼ tsp minced garlic
½ tsp ground cumin
½ tsp dry dill weed

½ cup vegan mayonnaise

Preparation

Break the tempeh into chunks and steam it over boiling water for 15 minutes. Set aside and allow to cool. Mix the rest of the ingredients in a bowl except the mayonnaise Crumble the tempeh into the bowl with the vegetables. Add the mayonnaise. Chill before serving. Makes 4 servings.

Teriyaki Tempeh Lettuce Wraps

Ingredients
1 diced bell pepper
½ diced onion
2 minced garlic cloves
½ block crumbled tempeh
3 diced baby Bella mushrooms
1 tablespoon peanut oil
1/6 cup teriyaki sauce
½ tsp sriracha
¼ tsp ginger paste

Preparation

Sauté the vegetables in oil until soft. Stir in the tempeh and heat completely. Add the teriyaki sauce and spices. Stir until blended. Serve on lettuce leaves. Makes 5 wraps.

Deli Tempeh Sandwich

Ingredients
4 oz tempeh
4 slices of whole grain bread
2 tsp soy sauce
½ tsp Herbes De Provence
Quick spray of canola oil
2 slices of tomato
2 Romaine lettuce leaves
2 oz sweet onion

2 oz vegan coleslaw
2 tablespoons vegan mayonnaise
2 tsp sweet relish
2 tablespoons vegan potato salad

Preparation

Add ½ of each ingredient on the whole grain bread. Top with the other slice of bread. Makes 2 servings.

Grilled Tempeh with Kiwi Salsa

Ingredients
12 oz block of tempeh
3 tablespoons soy sauce
1 tablespoon rice vinegar
¼ cup water
Tad of garlic powder
Tad of onion powder

For the kiwi salsa
4 chopped kiwis
1 chopped onion
1 chopped jalapeno
¼ cup chopped cilantro
Lime juice
1 tsp sugar
Salt & pepper to taste

Preparation

Mix the soy sauce, vinegar, water, garlic powder, and onion powder in a bowl. Place this marinade in a shallow baking dish. Slice the tempeh into thick locks. Add to the marinade and marinate for 30 minutes. Spray the grill with a touch of oil and put the tempeh slices on the grill. Cook until lightly browned.

Salsa

Peel and cut the kiwis into small pieces and place in a bowl. Sprinkle with 1 tsp of sugar and set aside. Chop the cilantro, jalapeno, and onion. Add to the kiwi. Sprinkle with lime juice and blend well. Salt and pepper to taste. Place the salsa on the side of the tempeh or on top. Makes 4 servings.

Chapter 6 - Dips & Spreads

Walnut Olive Spread

Ingredients

2 cups walnuts
1 1/3 cup black olives
½ cup parsley leaves
½ cup grated carrot
4 tablespoon nutritional yeast
4 tablespoon almond butter
2 tablespoon lime juice
Pepper to taste

Preparation

Soak the walnuts overnight in water. Drain and rinse the walnuts. In a food processor, place all ingredients except parsley, olives, and walnuts, process until finely chopped and clumping together. Add more butter as needed. Using a stick blender chop parsley, olives, and walnuts in small pieces. Add the ingredients to a pitcher and blend to a paste using a mixer. Makes 12 servings.

Avocado Dip

Ingredients

2 diced avocados
2 cans black beans (drained)
2 cans whole kernel corn (drained)
2 minced onions
1 ½ cups salsa
2 tablespoons chopped cilantro
2 tablespoons lemon juice
4 tablespoons chili powder
Salt and pepper to taste

Preparation

Samantha Michaels

Mix all ingredients expect the chili powder, salt and pepper in a bowl until well blended. Now add the left out ingredients. Makes 12 servings.

Sun-Dried Tomato Pesto

Ingredients

4 cups basil leaves
10 sun dried tomatoes
6 crushed garlic cloves
½ tsp salt
6 tablespoons toasted pine nuts
½ cup olive oil

Preparation

In a blender add the tomatoes, basil, nuts, salt, and garlic. Puree. Add the oil slowly and blend until desired texture. Makes 6 servings.

Cilantro Edamame Hummus

Ingredients

24 ounces of frozen green soybeans
4 garlic cloves
1 cup tahini
1 cup water
1 cup cilantro leaves
½ cup lemon juice
6 tablespoons olive oil
2 tsp kosher salt
1 ½ tsp ground cumin
¼ tsp cayenne pepper

Preparation

Add the soybeans in a large pot and cover with salted water. Cook over medium low heat until it begins to simmer. Cook until tender around 5 minutes. Drain. Puree the garlic in a food processor until minced. Add the cumin, salt, lemon juice, olive oil, cilantro, water, tahini, soybeans, and cayenne pepper. Blend until smooth. Makes 16 servings.

Veggie Pate

Ingredients

½ cup sunflower seeds
¼ cup whole wheat flour
¼ cup nutritional yeast
¼ tsp salt
¼ cup oil
1 tablespoon lemon juice
1 small chopped potato
1 small sliced carrot
1 small chopped onion
1 chopped celery stalk
1 garlic clove
¾ cup water
¼ tsp dried thyme
¼ tsp dried basil
¼ tsp dried sage
¼ tsp dried savory
¼ tsp black pepper
¼ tsp dry mustard

Preparation

Preheat oven to 350 degrees Fahrenheit. Grease a baking dish. Place all ingredients in a food processor and blend well. Process until almost smooth. Place the mixture in the baking dish. Bake for 1 hour. Makes 8 servings.

Five Pepper Hummus

Ingredients

1 small green bell pepper
8 oz drained garbanzo beans
2 jalapeno peppers
8 oz banana peppers
½ garlic clove

½ tablespoon ground cayenne pepper
1 tablespoons pepper
1/8 cup tahini

Preparation

Cut the top off the green bell pepper. Remove the seeds and pulp from both parts of the pepper. Chop part of the pepper and place in a blender with the jalapeno peppers, beans, banana peppers, cayenne pepper, garlic, tahini, and pepper. Blend until you have a smooth paste. Place in the green bell pepper and serve. Makes 8 servings.

Eggplant Antipasto

Ingredients

1 eggplant cubed
1 chopped onion
2 minced garlic cloves
1/3 cup chopped green bell pepper
3/4 cup sliced mushrooms
1/3 cup olive oil
¼ cup water
½ cup sliced stuffed green olives
1 tsp salt
6 oz tomato paste
2 tablespoons red wine vinegar
1 ½ tsp white sugar
¼ tsp dried basil
¼ tsp dried oregano
¼ tsp ground black pepper

Preparation

Preheat oven to 350 degrees Fahrenheit. In a baking dish, mix the bell pepper, olive oil, mushrooms, garlic, onion, and eggplant. Bake 10 minutes. Remove from oven and add water, tomato paste, salt, stuffed green olives, vinegar, basil, sugar, pepper, and oregano. Bake for another 30 minutes or until the eggplant is tender. Chill in the refrigerator for at least 8 hours before serving. Makes 48 servings.

Magaricz

Ingredients

½ cup olive oil
2 chopped eggplant
2 red bell peppers cut into strips
2 green bell peppers cut into strips
2 diced onions
2 cups shredded carrots
Crushed red pepper flakes
Salt to taste

Preparation

Place the eggplant in a colander. Lightly salt and leave to drain for 45 minutes. Heat the oil in a large skillet. Add the peppers, onion, carrot, and eggplant. Stir to coat in the oil. Reduce heat to low and cook 40 minutes stirring once in awhile until the mixture resembles jam. Season to taste. Cover and chill for 1 hour. Makes 20 servings.

Spicy Bean Dip

Ingredients

2 cups cooked pinto beans
2 cups hot salsa
2 tablespoons lime juice
2 tsp ground coriander
4 tsp ground cumin
½ tsp salt
Tad of cayenne

Preparation

Blend the beans until smooth in a blender. Add the coriander, lime juice, salsa, cumin, cayenne, pepper, and salt. Blend well. Pour into a bowl and garnish with parsley. Makes 8 servings.

Samantha Michaels

Cashew Mayonnaise

Ingredients

½ cup cashew pieces
1/8 cup water
1/8 cup lemon juice
1 soft date
½ tsp salt
½ tsp onion powder
¼ tsp garlic powder
1 tablespoon extra virgin olive oil
1 tablespoon flaxseed oil

Preparation

Combine in a blender the water, cashews, date, lemon juice, onion powder, salt, pepper, and garlic powder. Process until smooth. Keep the blender going and add the flaxseed oil and olive oil in a steam until emulsified. Makes 8 servings.

MORE 70 BEST EVER RECIPES EBOOKS REVEALED AT MY AUTHOR PAGE:-

CLICK HERE TO ACCESS THEM NOW

Printed in Great Britain
by Amazon